Home Remedies
For Worms

Home Remedies
For Worms

By Monica Sidoine,
S.N.H.S. Dip. Herbalism

DISCLAIMER

This book is to serve as an informational guide for use in the home. The remedies and procedures contained in this book are meant to supplement and are not intended to be a substitute for professional medical care. Please seek a qualified medical practitioner for all ailments. The author nor distributors takes no responsibility for customers choosing to treat themselves. Your use of this information is at your own risk.

Copyright © 2016
By
Monica Sidoine

ISBN - 13: 978-1535347723
ISBN - 10: 1535347724

Proof Read by Jasmine Ned Anunda

Printed By Create Space Publishing
United States of America

ACKNOWLEDGMENTS

I would like to thank all those who have contributed in one way or another to the completion of HOME REMEDIES FOR WORMS.

I thank God for giving me the vision, wisdom and good health to write this book. For all he has done and will continue to do in my life.

For the many prayer warriors who interceded on behalf of this project and also their moral support.

I thank my daughter Jasmine Ned Anunda for proof reading.

Thank you all.

Monica Sidoine.

PREFACE

The procedures in this Book was designed to be as simple as possible so that anyone will be able to follow them. Most of the items used are local things which you would either have at home, in your kitchen garden or can be easily purchased from the local market or health store for a very low cost.

By using the simple remedies and health tips outlined in this book it should help you in your journey to recovery.

TABLE OF CONTENTS

WORMS

What is worms?
Worms is an infestation of parasites, especially pinworms or tapeworms, affecting the intestines or other parts of a person's or animal's body. They live in the gastrointestinal tract or they dig through it into the muscles. They also eat your food.

What can it cause?
It can cause anemia.
It can cause diarrhea.
It can cause gas and bloating.
It can cause weight loss.
It can cause loss of appetite.
It can cause malnutrition.
It can cause rectal prolapse.
It can cause itching around the anal area.
It can affect the mental function.
It can cause reactions in the tissues.
It can cause you to be sick.
It can also affect the absorption of nutrients in the body.
They produce toxic waste in your body.

How is it transmitted?
It is transmitted by persons passing out the worm eggs in their feces onto the soil or into the water.
Then persons partaking of contaminated food and drink which have the eggs.
Also by the worm entering the skin as a result of walking barefoot on infected soil.

NATURAL REMEDIES

- Crush 7-14oz of pumpkin seeds for children and up to 25oz for adults. Stir it into fruit juice to make a pulp to be eaten. Consume it and 2 or 3 hours later take 2 tablespoons of castor oil to expel the worms.

- Crush 1 cup of soursop seeds into a powder. Mix it with 1 cup of milk, water or fruit juice. Consume it.

- Dry 1 cup of papaya seeds and crush it to a powder. Mix it with 1 cup of milk or water. Drink half of it twice daily, the last one 2 hours after supper. **N.B. Dosage may be repeated after 1 week if needed.**

- Collect 3-4 teaspoons of milk from a green papaya fruit or from the trunk of the tree when it is cut. Mix it with an equal amount of sugar and stir it into a cup of hot water. It can also be drank with a laxative.

- Steep 1oz of papaya leaves in 1 liter of boiling water for 30 minutes. Drink 1 cup 3 times daily.

- Steep 1oz of lemon grass or 9 leaves in 1 liter of boiling water for 30 minutes. It can be sweetened with honey. Drink 1 cup 4 times daily.

- Steep 1oz of chamomile in 1 liter of boiling water for 20 minutes. Drink 1 cup 4 times daily.

- Steep 1oz of rosemary leaves in 1 liter of boiling water for 30 minutes.
  Drink 1 cup 4 times daily.

- Steep 1oz of tamarind leaves in 1 liter of boiling water for 30 minutes.
  Drink 1 cup 3 times daily.

- Steep 1oz of ginger in 1 liter of boiling water for 20 minutes.
  Drink 1 cup 4 times daily.

- Steep 1oz of turmeric in 1 liter of boiling water for 20 minutes.
  Drink 1 cup 4 times daily.

- Steep 1oz of cloves in 1 liter of boiling water for 30 minutes.
  Drink 1 cup 4 times daily.

- Boil a garlic bulb in 1 liter of water for 5 minutes.
  Drink 1 cup 3 times daily.

- Boil 8 mashed avocado seeds until it becomes like a light paste and strain it.
  Drink ½ cup three times daily.

- Blend one onion, 1½ glasses of lemon or carrot juice.
  Take half a glass by spoonfuls three times daily.

- Blend 3 garlic cloves and 6oz carrot juice.
  Take it every two hours daily.

- Take 2 glasses of pomegranate juice daily.

- Take 2 glasses of figs juice daily.

- Drink ¼ cup of aloe 3 times daily.

- Eat grapefruit and soursop fruit daily.

- Eat 3 slices of ripe pineapple with each meal for 1 week.

- Eat 2 bitter lemons each day for 7-10 days.

- Eat 2lbs of grated carrot daily as a meal or 2 carrots for breakfast for a week.

- Eat five raw garlic cloves and raw onions with each meal.

- Insert a clove of garlic into the anus.

- Take an Epsom Salt Bath.

EPSOM SALT BATH

Procedure:

1. Pour 1-2lb of Epsom salt into a tub of hot water.
2. While soaking in it for 30 minutes drink 2-3 cups of hot herbal tea.

Immediately after the bath rest and cover warmly so profuse sweating can begin.

- **N.B. When pinworms come out at night.**
  Soak a cotton with oil and use it to remove the pinworm. Change the bed sheet, underwear and pajamas each night for 1 week.

HEALTH TIPS

- If you are eating watercress, make sure that it is properly washed, since it grows in streams, if it is polluted there is a possibility that it might be contaminated with worms.

- Make sure that you wash all foods which you will be eating raw very well.

- If you have to use water from a polluted source for drinking purposes, boil it before using it.

- Wash your hands as often as possible especially before each meal and after using the restroom.

- Wash all clothing items in very hot soapy water as often as possible.

- Avoid walking barefoot.

- Use the toilet to pass your feces not on the ground.

- Be careful of getting in contact with the feces of other persons.

- Be aware of the symptoms and if you notice them, try to act on it as soon as possible.

GUINEA WORMS

This is a long thin worm which lives under the skin of humans and animals.
It can grow to about 3 feet long.
They can lay thousands of eggs.
Sometimes you can have it over a span of 1 year without knowing, not until the sore develops and the adult worm comes out to lay its eggs.

Symptoms:
Swelling accompanied with lots of pain occurring most times in the legs, testicles and ankles.
About 1 week after that, a blister appears and it turns into a sore.

Causes:
Drinking water which has been infected by it.
Bathing or walking in pools which have been infected.
If someone who is already infected with it have an open sore and goes into water, the worm puts it's head out and lays eggs into the water.

NATURAL REMEDIES

- Make sure that the sore is properly cleaned. Keep it soaked in cold water until you see the head of the worm comes out. Tie a string to it and each day gently ease it out a little at a time. Being very careful not to break it.

- **If an infection develops:**
  Steep 1oz ginger in 1 liter of boiling water for 20 minutes.
  Drink 1 cup 4 times daily.

- Steep 1oz of thyme in 1 liter of boiling water for 20 minutes. Drink 1 cup 4 times daily.

- Steep 1oz of rosemary in 1 liter of boiling water for 20 minutes. Drink 1 cup 4 times daily.

- Eat 3 cloves of raw grated garlic 3 times daily.

HEALTH TIPS

- Boil all water which will be used for drinking.

- Avoid using contaminated water.

- Avoid drinking water from the pool.

HOOKWORM

They are normally red and about ½ inch long.

Symptoms are:
Nausea, vomiting, diarrhea and stomach ache.
Anemia and protein deficiency after the infection.

Other symptoms that might be possible:
Cramps.
Loss of appetite.

Shortness of breath.
Heart failure.
Mucus in the stools.
Bloody or dark stools.
Swelling in the legs and of the body.
Incontinence in men.

How is it transmitted?
From pets.
Through contaminated food and water.
If the feces gets in contact with the soil and you walk on it barefoot, if you don't wash your hands before eating, it can enter in through the skin.

NATURAL REMEDIES

- Steep 1oz of turmeric in 1 liter of boiling water for 20 minutes.
  Drink 1 cup 4 times daily.

- Steep 1oz thyme in 1 liter of boiling water for 20 minutes.
  Drink 1 cup 4 times daily.

- Collect 3-4 teaspoons of milk from a green papaya fruit or the trunk of the tree when it is cut. Mix it with an equal amount of sugar and stir it into a cup of hot water.
  It can also be drank with a laxative.

- Eat 6 teaspoons of grated raw garlic daily.

- Eat carrots daily as part of your diet.

- Eat ¼ cup of pumpkin seeds daily.

- Chew 2 cloves twice daily.

- Use thyme in your cooking.

- Consume 3 tablespoons of coconut oil and 1 glass of coconut water daily. Massage the area with coconut oil.

HEALTH TIPS

- Wear shoes at all times especial when going outdoors.

- Use the toilets at all times.

PINWORMS

They are thin and white, about ½" long. They lay their eggs outside of the anus which can be in the thousands.

The symptoms are:
Rectal itching especially at nights.
Mild abdominal pain.

Causes are:
Eating raw vegetables. Consuming vegetables which are not properly cooked.
Inhaling dust from homes were pets also reside with humans.

How is it transmitted?
It can be transmitted through the infected person scratching their anus, and the eggs getting stuck under their fingernails, which is then passed onto another person entering in through the mouth. The females travel to the outside of the anus during the night to deposit their eggs.

NATURAL REMEDIES

- Consume 3 tablespoons of coconut oil and 1 glass of coconut water daily. Massage the area with coconut oil.

- Blend 3 raw cloves of garlic and 1 cup of carrot juice. Drink it every 2 hours.

- Eat 2 bitter lemons each day for 10 days.

- Add 3 teaspoons of salt to ½ liter of water. Use it as an enema.

- **N.B. When pinworms come out at night.**
  Soak a cotton with oil and use it to remove the pinworm. Change the bed sheet and sleepwear each night for 1 week.

HEALTH TIPS

- Sleep alone.

- Wash your hands often, especially after every visit to the toilet and upon waking up.

- Wash your clothes and your bed linens as often as possible in hot soapy water.

- Bathe as often as possible paying special attention to the nails and anus.

- Just before bedtime put some Vaseline around the anus.

- Cut the fingernails very short.

- Avoid putting your fingers in your mouth.

- Avoid scratching your anus.

ROUNDWORMS (Ascaris)

Pink or white about 1 foot long. It is most common in tropical and subtropical areas.

Causes are:
Poor hygiene.
Contaminated food and water which have the eggs in them.
Human excretion which is being used as fertilizer.

Symptoms are:
Itching,
Coughing and maybe pneumonia with the coughing up of blood.
Diarrhea, indigestion, abdominal pains, weakness.
They may cause swollen bellies in children.

The eggs are passed via the feces and then taken in orally. They hatch and enter the bloodstream, then travel to the lungs, the young ones are coughed up and then swallowed and this is where they will grow to a full size in the intestine.

NATURAL REMEDIES

- Drink 2 glasses of coconut water daily.

- Steep 1oz of neem in 1 liter of boiling water for 20 minutes. Drink 1 cup 4 times daily.

- Steep 1oz of turmeric in 1 liter of boiling water for 20 minutes. Drink 1 cup 4 times daily.

- Steep 1oz of bamboo leaves in 1 liter of boiling for 30 minutes. Drink 1 cup 4 times daily.

- Steep 1oz of hyssop in 1 liter of boiling water for 20 minutes. Drink 1 cup 4 times daily.

- Soak 4 chopped raw onions in 1 liter of water for 12 hours. Squeeze the onions and strain it. Drink 1 cup 4 times daily. Do a garlic enema along with it.

- Blend 3 garlic cloves and 1 cup of carrot juice. Drink it every 2 hours.

- Dry 1 cup of papaya seeds and crush it to a powder. Mix it with 1 cup of milk or water.
  Drink half of it twice daily, the last one 2 hours after supper. Do it for 1 week.
  N.B. Dosage may be repeated after 1 week if needed

- Collect 3-4 teaspoons of milk from a green papaya fruit or the trunk of the tree when it is cut. Mix it with an equal amount of sugar and stir it into a cup of hot water.
  Drink it. It can also be drank with a laxative.

- Eat pomegranate.

- Eat carrots daily.

- Eat 5 raw garlic cloves 3 times daily.

- Use thyme in your cooking.

- Use the same remedy as for worms.

HEALTH TIPS

- Use toilets at all times, do not do it on the ground.

- Make sure that your hands and fingernails are washed very clean before eating or handling food items.

- Cover all foodstuffs.

TAPEWORMS

There are three kinds of tapeworms:
Beef Tapeworm, Fish Tapeworm and Pork Tapeworm.

The most common are Beef and Pork Tapeworm.
Blindness and epilepsy can occur as a result of Pork Tapeworm.

The worms are flat segmented and can mature to 20-30 feet while they are in the intestines. Most times they are passed out in pieces which are normally filled with eggs.

Causes are:
By eating undercooked or raw meat or fish. In this case they will live in the intestines.
Ingesting the eggs through taking in contaminated food or water. In this case they will make cysts in the brain, muscles and tissues.
If they move from the intestine into the stomach.

Symptoms are:
If they are in the intestines:
Diarrhea.
Mild abdominal pain.
Malnutrition.

If they are in the cysts:
Seizures.
Meningitis.
Fluid accumulation in the brain.
Changes in the way you think.
They can also go into the spinal cord or the eye.

NATURAL REMEDIES

- Eat 2 ½ cups of dried coconut. Don't eat anything after it.
  Drink lots of water.
  Mix 1 tablespoon of Epsom salt with 1 cup of water.
  Drink it about 2 hours after your last meal.
  Drink a glass of water after it.
  Wait for about 2 hours and just before going to bed, drink
  another dosage of the Epsom salt.
  Drink a glass of water after it.
  N.B. This treatment will purge you.

- Take 2 tablespoons of castor oil.
  Only eat fruits or drink fruit juices for the next 24 hours.
  Crush ¼ cup of pumpkin seeds and add 1 tablespoon of
  honey to it.
  Consume it.
  After 1 hour take 4 tablespoons of castor oil.
  After 3 hours take an enema using 1 liter of fluid.
  **N.B. Try not to vomit the contents of the treatment. You
  might have a loose bowel movement.
  If the worm doesn't come out. Repeat the treatment at
  some other time.**

- Drink 2 glasses of coconut water daily.

- Steep 1oz of neem in 1 liter of boiling water for 20 minutes.
  Drink 1 cup 4 times daily.

- Steep 1oz of turmeric in 1 liter of boiling water for 20
  minutes.
  Drink 1 cup 4 times daily.

- Steep 1oz of bamboo leaves in 1 liter of boiling water for 30 minutes.
  Drink 1 cup 4 times daily.

- Steep 1oz of hyssop in 1 liter of boiling water for 20 minutes.
  Drink 1 cup 4 times daily.

- Go on a fast for 3 days only eating raw pineapple.

- Eat pomegranates.

- Eat carrots daily.

- Eat 3 raw garlic cloves 3 times daily.

HEALTH TIPS

- If you will be eating meat or fish, make sure that it is properly cooked.

TRICHINOSIS

It is caused by very small worms which can be hardly seen in the feces.

The symptoms are:
Diarrhea, abdominal cramps, nausea and stomach aches.

It can be acquired by:
Eating raw or uncooked pork.
Burrow from the intestines through the tissues of the body to the muscles and also the heart.

NATURAL REMEDIES

- See the same remedies for worms.

HEALTH TIP

- Avoid eating raw or uncooked pork.

WHIPWORMS

They are 1-2 inches long and either pink or grey.

Symptoms are:
Diarrhea.
Prolapse of the rectum.

It is transmitted from feces to the mouth.

NATURAL REMEDIES

- See the same remedies for worms.

- **If there is a prolapse of the rectum:**
Turn the child upside down and pour cool water on the intestine to help it go back inside.

HEALTH TIPS

- Wash your hands very well after every bowel movement.

- Avoid putting your hands to your mouth if they are dirty.

Other Book Titles by the Same Author

Can be viewed at this link:
http://www.amazon.com/author/monicasidoine

Healing Poultices

The Top 20 Most Valuable Herbs

Home Remedies For Cancer

Home Remedies For Eczema

Home Remedies For Losing Weight

Home Remedies For Blood Pressure and Diabetes

Home Remedies For Headaches and Insomnia

Home Remedies For Sinusitis and Tonsillitis

Home Remedies For Constipation and Diarrhea

Home Remedies For Asthma and Bronchitis

Home Remedies For Dehydration and Vomiting

Home Remedies For Pneumonia and Tuberculosis

Home Remedies For Stress, Depression and Anxiety

Home Remedies For Dengue and Malaria

Home Remedies For Heart Attack and Strokes

Home Remedies For Colds, Fever and Sore Throat

NOTES

NOTES

NOTES

NOTES